Recipes for an Alkaline Diet

Maintaining your Bodies pH is The Key to Health and Longevity

By

Jennifer Jones

License Notices

Get Your Daily Deals Here!

Thanks for buying my book! As a special offer, you are now eligible for free books when you sign up below. All you need to do is fill in your email address and offers will be emailed to you on a daily basis for free and discounted books. To make sure you never miss one of these unique offers, a reminder email will be sent to you a few days before the offer expires. You don't have to do a thing! Subscribe now in the box below and start receiving your thank you gift!

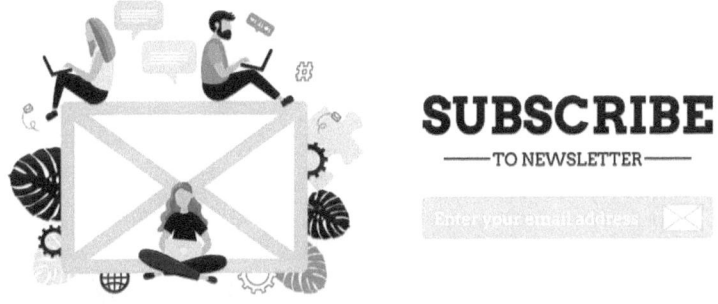

SUBSCRIBE

—— TO NEWSLETTER ——

Enter your email address

https://Jennifer-Jones.gr8.com

Table of Contents

Alkaline Diet Recipes

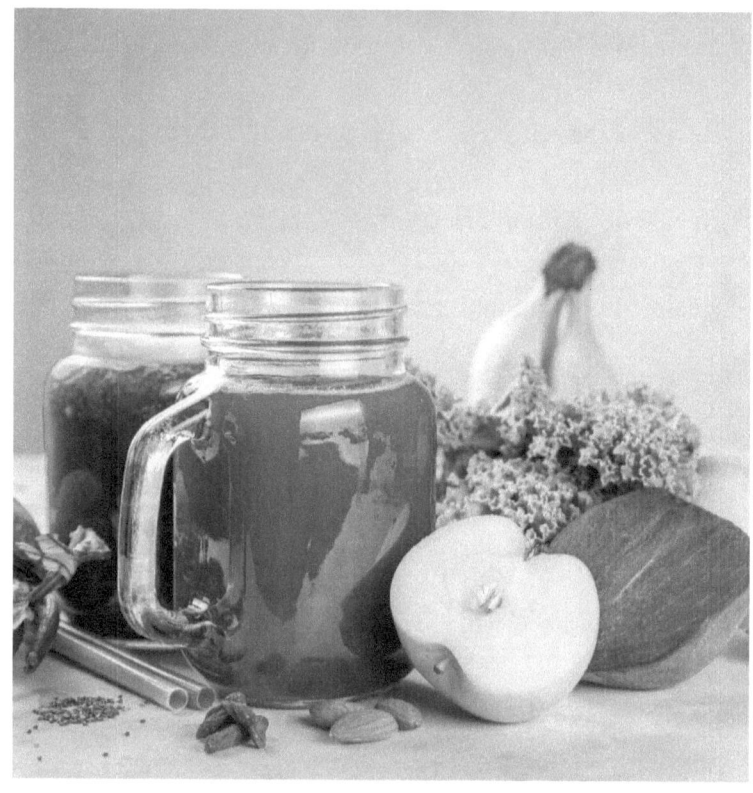

HHHHHHHHHHHHHHHHHHHHHHHHHHHHHHHHHHHHHHHHHH

Recipe 1: Mustard Greens and Butter Beans

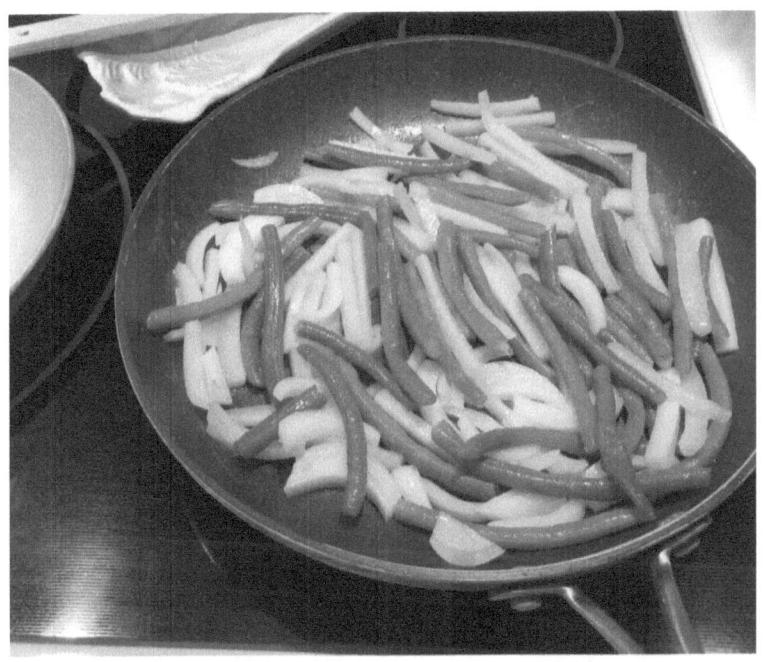

Mustard greens are a great source of iron!

Serving Size: 4 servings

Ingredient List:

- 2 cups cooked mustard greens
- 2 cups cooked butter beans
- ½ Tablespoons chopped rosemary
- 4 cup water or vegetable broth

HHHHHHHHHHHHHHHHHHHHHHHHHHHHHHHHHHHHHH

Procedure:

1. In Dutch oven combine: broth, mustard greens, beans, rosemary; stir; bring to boil, reduce heat, let simmer 10-15 minutes

Recipe 2: Alkaline Trail Mix

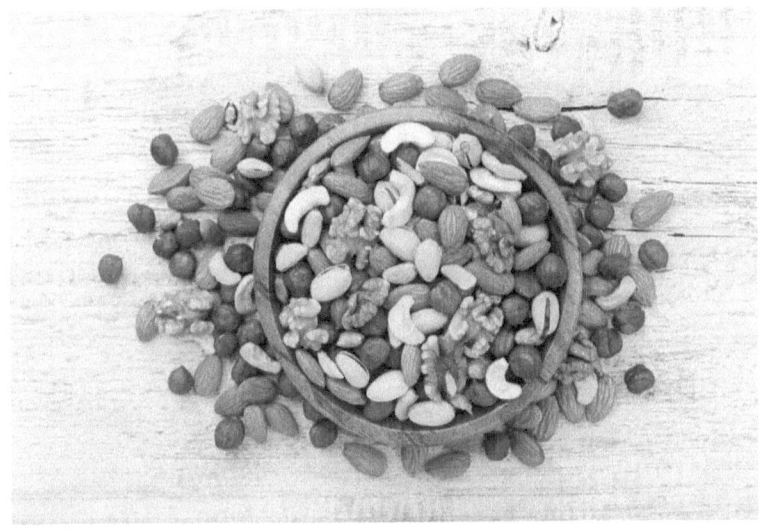

The perfect on the go snack!

Serving Size: approx.. 3-4 cups worth

Ingredient List:

- ¼ cup EACH: almonds, cashews, and pistachios
- 1/3 cup sunflower seeds
- 1/3 cup EACH: dried apricots, dried cranberries
- 1/3 cup raisins
- ½ cup candy coated chocolate pieces
- 1 cup bran flakes or honey oat cereal (ex. Cheerio's)

HHHHHHHHHHHHHHHHHHHHHHHHHHHHHHHHHHHHHH

Procedure:

1. Mix together almonds, cashews, pistachios, dried apricots, dried cranberries, raisins, candy coated pieces, cereal

Recipe 3: Chicken Wrap

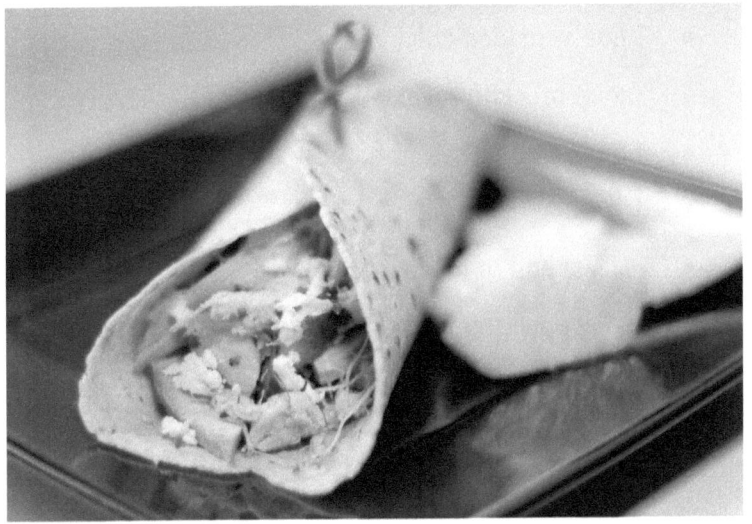

Ingredient List:

- 1 tablespoon olive oil
- 1 cup shredded chicken
- ½ cup broccoli pieces
- 4 quartered cherry tomatoes
- drizzle with lemon juice
- ½ teaspoon of celery salt
- ½ teaspoon thyme

HHHHHHHHHHHHHHHHHHHHHHHHHHHHHHHHHHHHHHH

Procedure:

1. In skillet over medium high heat and oil brown chicken, broccoli, tomato; top with celery, lemon juice, thyme; spoon into wrap

Recipe 4: Avocado Salsa

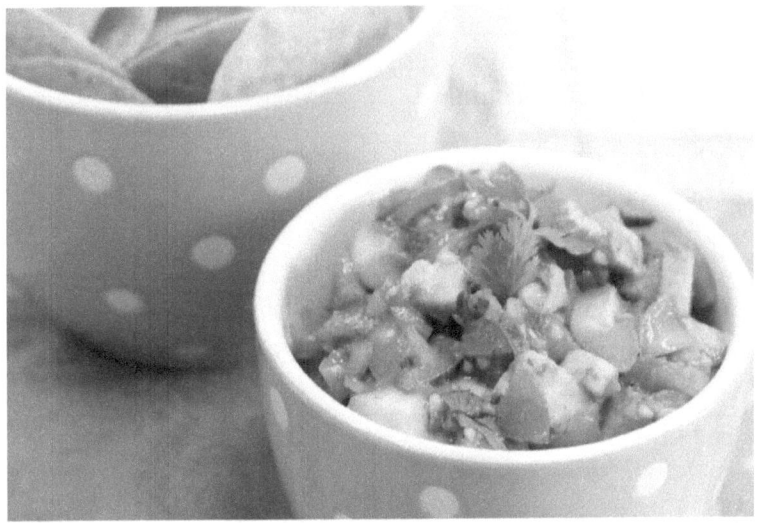

Great on lean proteins or with beans!

Serving Size: approx.. 2 cups

Ingredient List:

- 1 diced avocado
- ½ cucumber diced
- ½ diced zucchini
- ½ stalk of leek or bok choy diced
- Juice of 1 lemon
- 1 teaspoon cilantro (optional)

HHHHHHHHHHHHHHHHHHHHHHHHHHHHHHHHHHHHHHH

Procedure:

1. Mix together diced avocado, cucumber, zucchini, leek or bok choy and cilantro; pour lemon juice over them

Recipe 5: Tangy Morning Drink

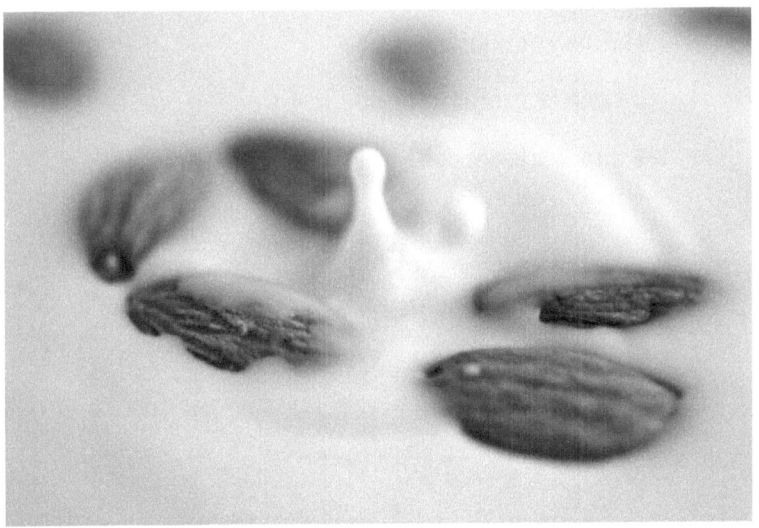

Great protein drink for mornings!

Serving Size: 1 serving

Ingredient List:

- 1 cup almond milk
- 1 tablespoon cherry juice
- 1/3 cup watermelon juice
- ½ cup watercress

HHHHHHHHHHHHHHHHHHHHHHHHHHHHHHHHHHHHHHHH

Procedure:

1. Blend almond milk, cherry juice, watermelon juice, watercress

Recipe 6: Rosemary, Egg, and Cheese Chips

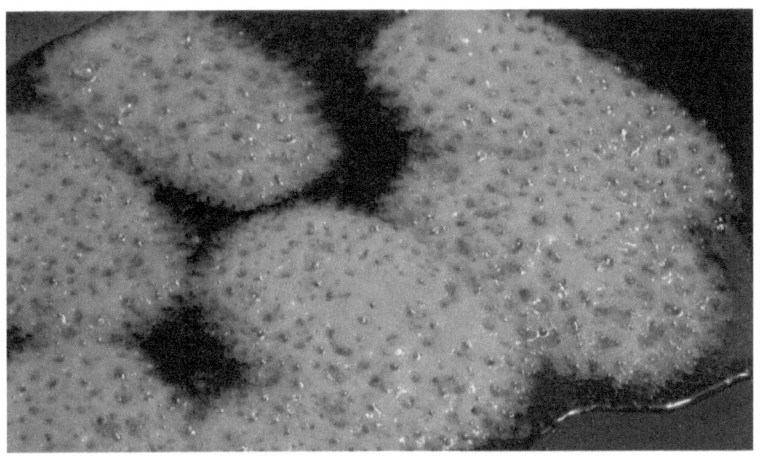

For when you feel like cutting loose!

Serving Size: 24 chips

Ingredient List:

- 3 egg whites
- 1/3 cup crumbled feta cheese or similar crumbled cheese
- ½ teaspoons onion powder or garlic powder (optional
- ½ teaspoons diced rosemary
- Coconut oil

HHHHHHHHHHHHHHHHHHHHHHHHHHHHHHHHHHHHHHHH

Procedure:

1. Preheat oven to 400 and prepare with coconut oil mini muffin pan

2. Combine: egg whites, cheese, spices, herbs; place small amount in each mini muffin slot; bake 15-20 minutes

Recipe 7: Kiwi Ginger Tea

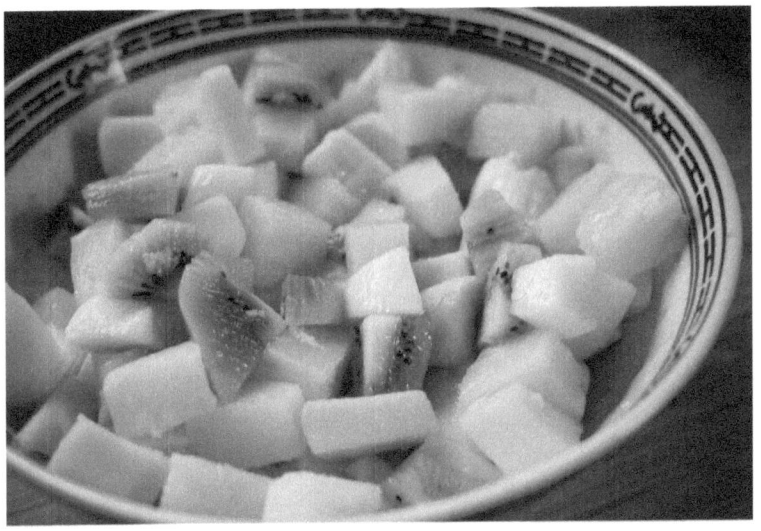

A great midday boost!

Serving Size: 1 serving

Ingredient List:

- 1-2 ginger tea bags
- 1 tablespoon honey
- Juice of 1 kiwi
- ¼ cup lemon juice

HHHHHHHHHHHHHHHHHHHHHHHHHHHHHHHHHHHHHH

Procedure:

1. Make tea, add honey, kiwi juice, lemon juice; stir and enjoy

Recipe 8: Lentil Soup

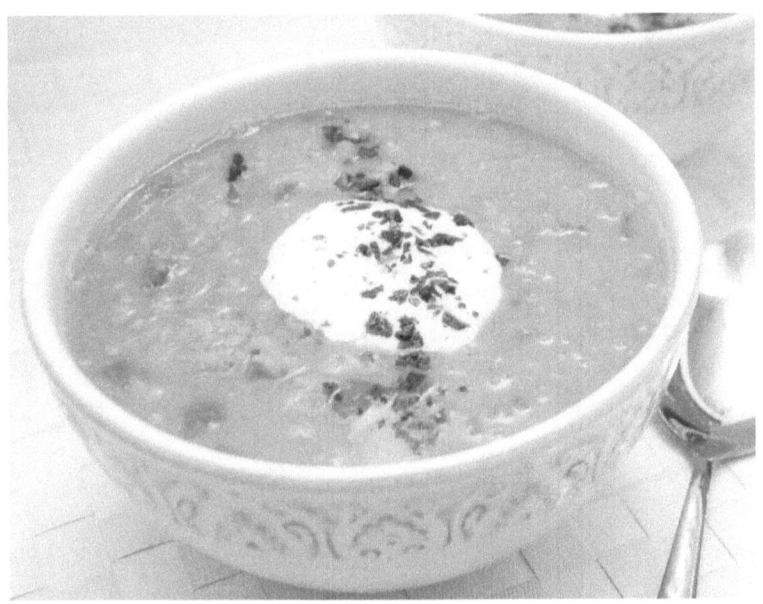

Perfect hardy lunch!

Serving Size: 4 servings.

Ingredient List:

- 4 cups vegetable broth
- 2 cups cooked lentils
- 1 cup peas
- 12-15 basil leaves

HHHHHHHHHHHHHHHHHHHHHHHHHHHHHHHHHHHHHHHH

Procedure:

1. In Dutch oven combine: broth, lentils, peas, basil; bring to boil, reduce heat, let simmer 10-15 minutes

Recipe 9: Lemon Melon Juice

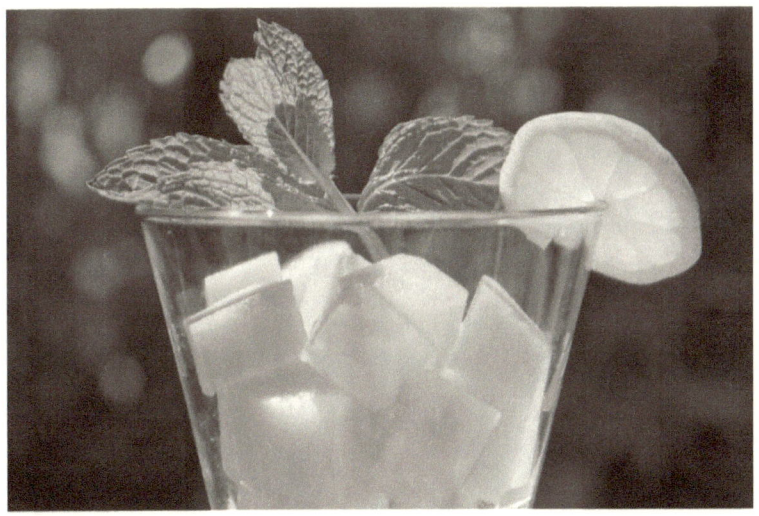

Mix it up and try in season melons!

Serving Size: 1 serving

Ingredient List:

- 1 cup watermelon juice
- ½ cup lemon juice
- 1 teaspoon honey

HHHHHHHHHHHHHHHHHHHHHHHHHHHHHHHHHHHHHHHH

Procedure:

1. Blend together watermelon juice, lemon juice, honey

Recipe 10: Pumpkin Soup

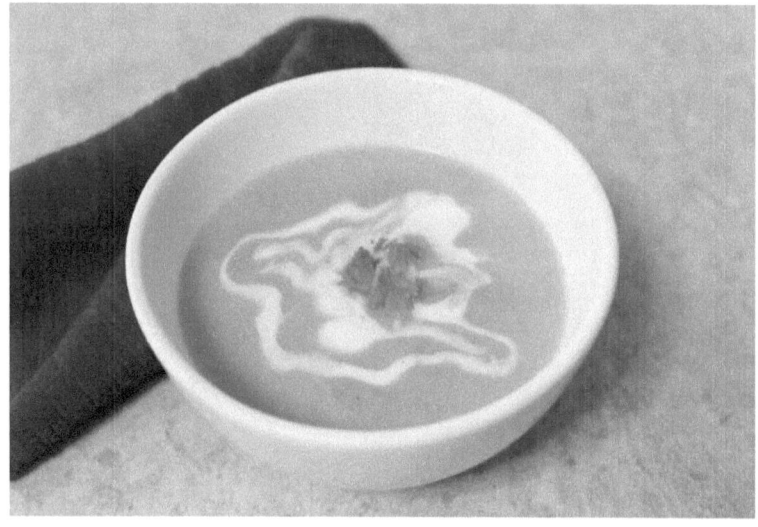

Add black or butter beans for texture!

Serving Size: 3 servings

Ingredient List:

- The flesh of 1 large pumpkin
- 2 cups diced leeks
- ½ cup parsley leaves
- 4 cups vegetable broth

HHHHHHHHHHHHHHHHHHHHHHHHHHHHHHHHHHHHHHH

Procedure:

1. Puree pumpkin flesh, add it along with diced leeks, parsley flowers, and broth; stir, bring to boil, reduce heat, let simmer 10-15 minutes

Recipe 11: Lavender Mint Tea

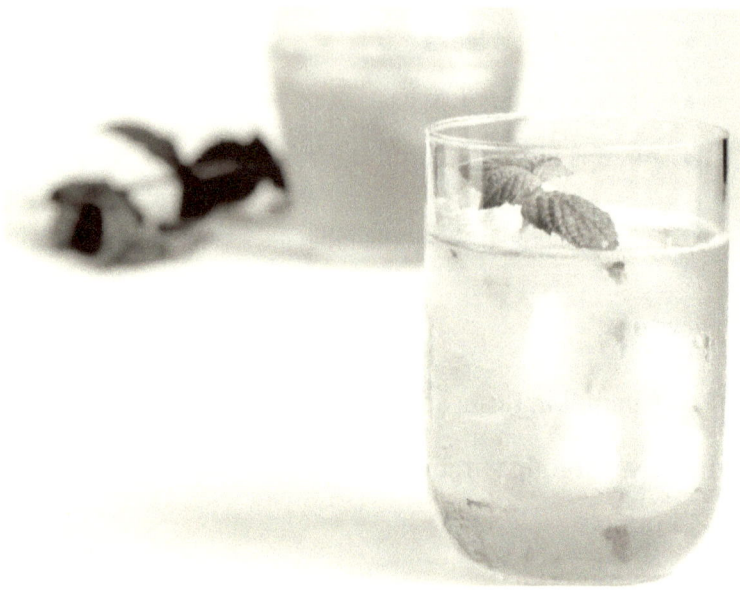

Ingredient List:

- 1 cup lavender tea
- 4-5 torn mint leaves
- ½ Tablespoons honey

HHHHHHHHHHHHHHHHHHHHHHHHHHHHHHHHHHHHHHHH

Procedure:

1. Blend together lavender tea, mint leaves, honey; serve hot or cold

Recipe 12: Quinoa Salad

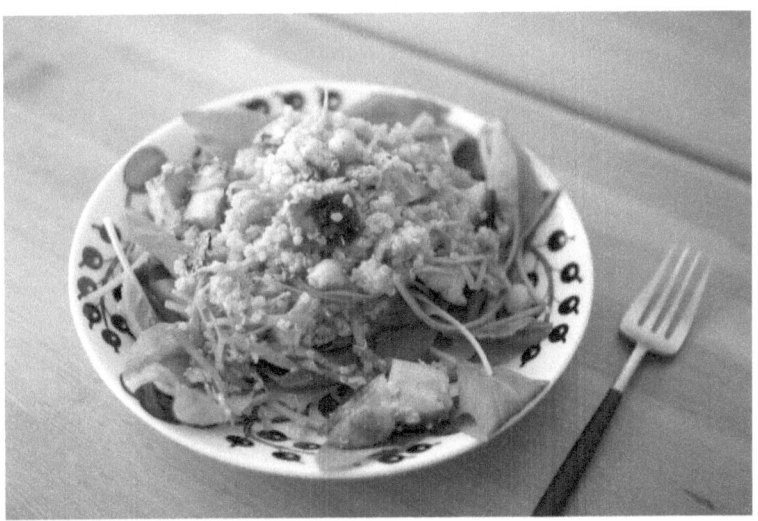

Great cold or hot!

Serving Size: approx. 2 cups

Ingredient List:

- 1 cup quinoa
- 2 cups alkaline water
- 1 cup grated broccoli
- 1 cup grated cabbage
- 1 cup chopped kale
- 8 quartered cherry tomatoes
- Juice of 1 lemon

HHHHHHHHHHHHHHHHHHHHHHHHHHHHHHHHHHHHHHH

Procedure:

1. Let quinoa sit in water until it has soaked it up; cook 8-10 minutes; stir in broccoli, cabbage, kale, tomatoes; pour in juice and stir well

Recipe 13: Cherry Almond Smoothie

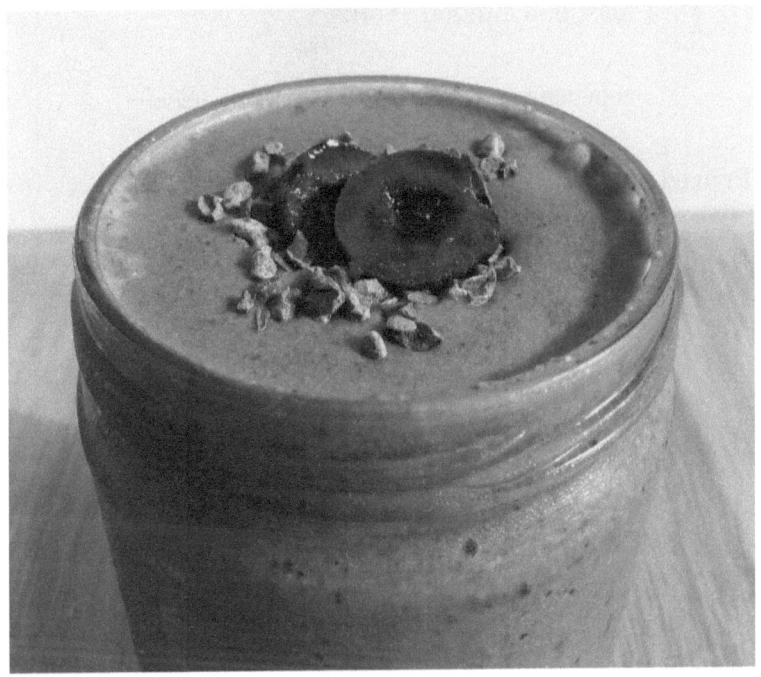

Add cherry juice if it is too "almondy" for you!

Serving Size: 1 serving

Ingredient List:

- 1 cup cherry vanilla yogurt
- 1 cup almond milk
- 1 teaspoon almond vanilla

HHHHHHHHHHHHHHHHHHHHHHHHHHHHHHHHHHHHHH

Procedure:

1. Blend together yogurt, almond milk, almond vanilla

Recipe 14: Onion Patties

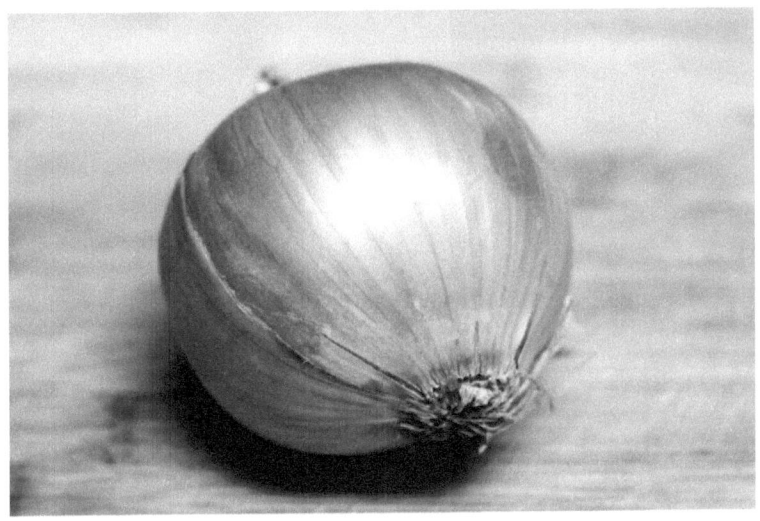

Great with kale added in!

Serving Size: 5 patties

Ingredient List:

- 1 cup almond flour
- 1 cup almond milk
- 1 cup chopped onion
- 1 teaspoon smoked paprika
- 1 teaspoon thyme or rosemary

HHHHHHHHHHHHHHHHHHHHHHHHHHHHHHHHHHHHHHH

Procedure:

1. Combine: flour, milk, onions, paprika, herbs; press into 1-2 thick patties and cook in skillet with coconut oil 4-6 minutes per side or until golden brown

Recipe 15: Pine Berry Juice

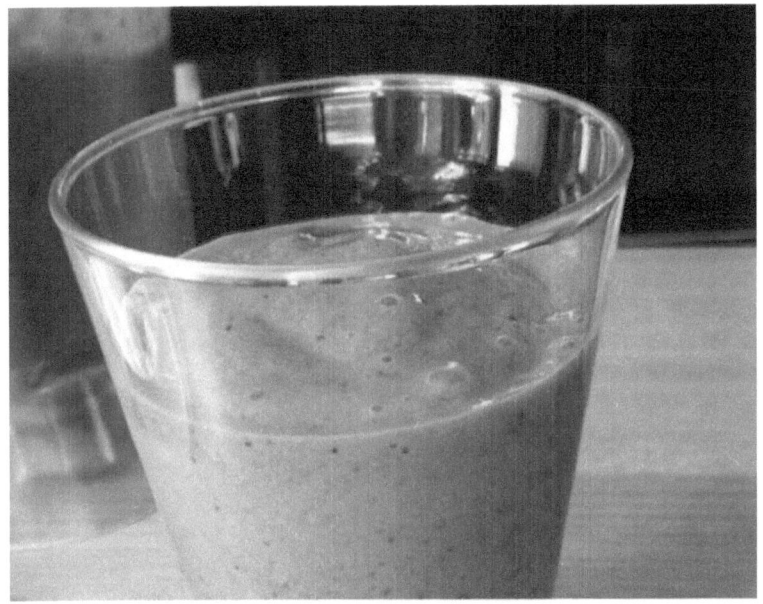

Try adding some ginger!

Serving Size: 1 serving

Ingredient List:

- ½ Tablespoons ginger juice
- ½ cup strawberries
- ⅓ cup pineapple juice

HHHHHHHHHHHHHHHHHHHHHHHHHHHHHHHHHHHHHHHH

Procedure:

1. Blend together ginger juice, strawberries, pineapple juice

Recipe 16: Coconut Hummus

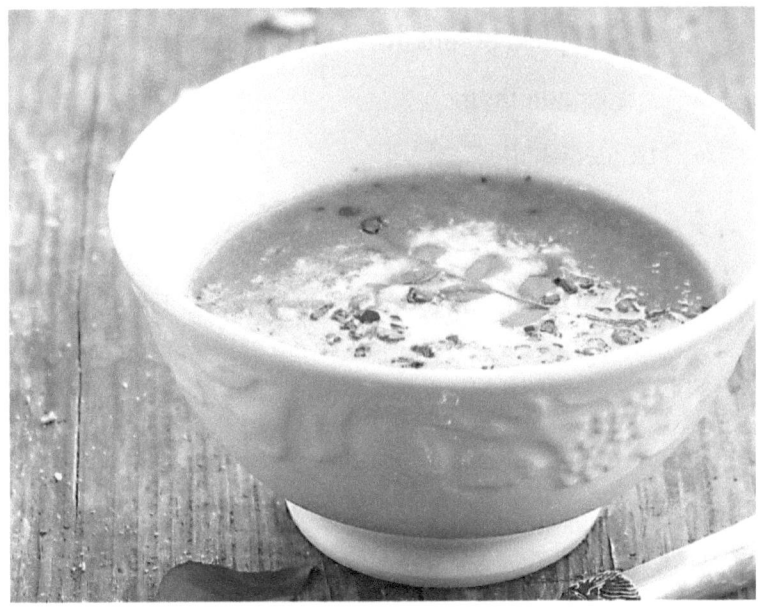

Great dip for roasted veggies!

Serving Size: approx. 2 cups

Ingredient List:

- 1 can, washed and drained, garbanzo beans
- 2/3 chopped pumpkin
- 1 teaspoon thyme
- 1 diced shallot
- ½ cup coconut flakes

HHHHHHHHHHHHHHHHHHHHHHHHHHHHHHHHHHHHHHHHHH

Procedure:

1. In blender puree beans, pumpkin, thyme; stir in diced shallot and coconut flakes

Recipe 17: Chocolate Coconut Smoothie

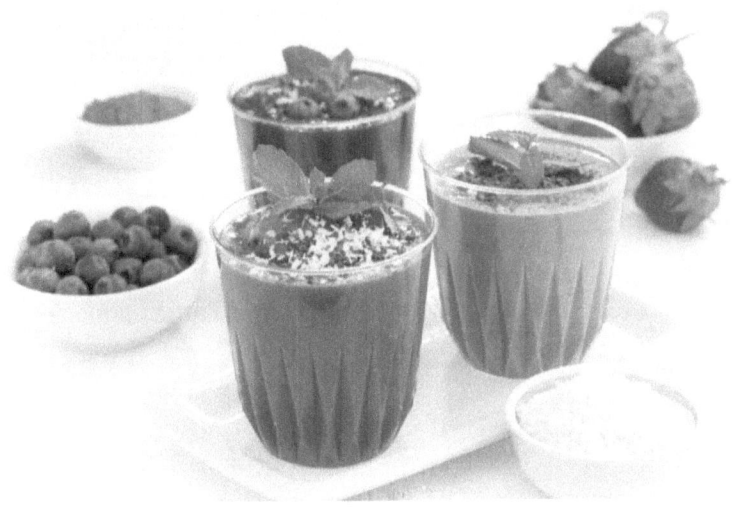

Great "pick me up" during meals and snacks!

Serving Size: 1 serving

Ingredient List:

- ¼ cup chocolate protein powder
- 1 cup plain yogurt
- ½ cup coconut milk
- ¼ cup cherry juice (optional)

HHHHHHHHHHHHHHHHHHHHHHHHHHHHHHHHHHHHHHH

Procedure:

1. Blend together protein powder, yogurt, milk, and cherry juice

Recipe 18: Celery, Onion, and Garlic Sauté

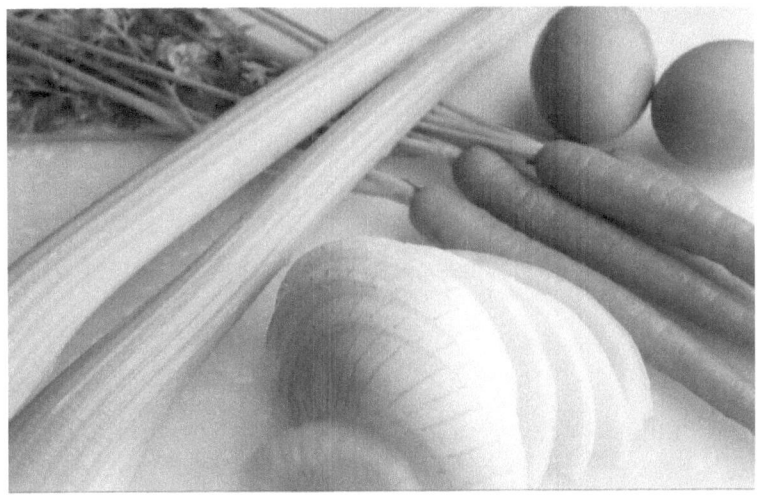

Use as a salsa!

Serving Size: approx. 2 cups

Ingredient List:

- 1 cup diced celery
- 1 diced onion
- 1 tablespoon diced or minced garlic
- ½ block cubed and firm tofu (optional)
- 1 cup almond flour
- Coconut oil for frying or sautéing

HHHHHHHHHHHHHHHHHHHHHHHHHHHHHHHHHHHHHHH

Procedure:

1. Combine: celery, onion, garlic, tofu, and flour; toss together; cook in skillet with coconut oil

Recipe 19: No Bake Cookies and Cream Protein Bars

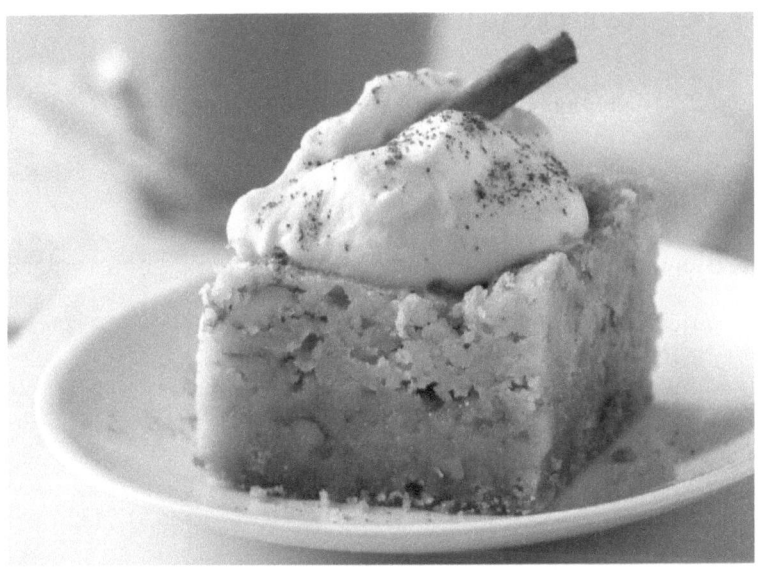

A high protein treats!

Serving Size: a 9x9 dish

Ingredient List:

- 1 cup cookies and cream protein powder
- 6 protein bars with nuts and chocolate
- 1 container vanilla Greek yogurt

HHHHHHHHHHHHHHHHHHHHHHHHHHHHHHHHHHHHHHHH

Procedure:

1. Blend together protein powder, protein bars, yogurt; place in a 9x9 dish and freeze 3 hours

Recipe 20: Cucumber Boats

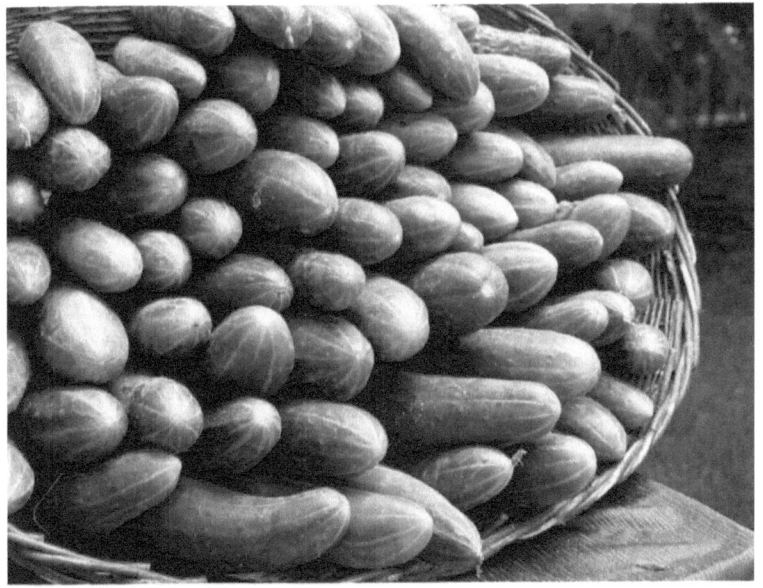

For add protein serve with Salmon!

Serving Size: 4 boats

Ingredient List:

- 4 cucumbers with centers dug out
- ½ cup diced roasted butternut squash
- ½ cup diced avocado
- 1 can, drained and washed, garbanzo or black beans
- 1 diced red onion
- 2 teaspoons EACH: diced oregano, diced rosemary
- ¼ cup coconut oil

HHHHHHHHHHHHHHHHHHHHHHHHHHHHHHHHHHHHHHHH

Procedure:

1. Combine: squash, avocado, beans, onion, herbs, oil; spoon into cucumbers

Recipe 21: Peary Kale Juice

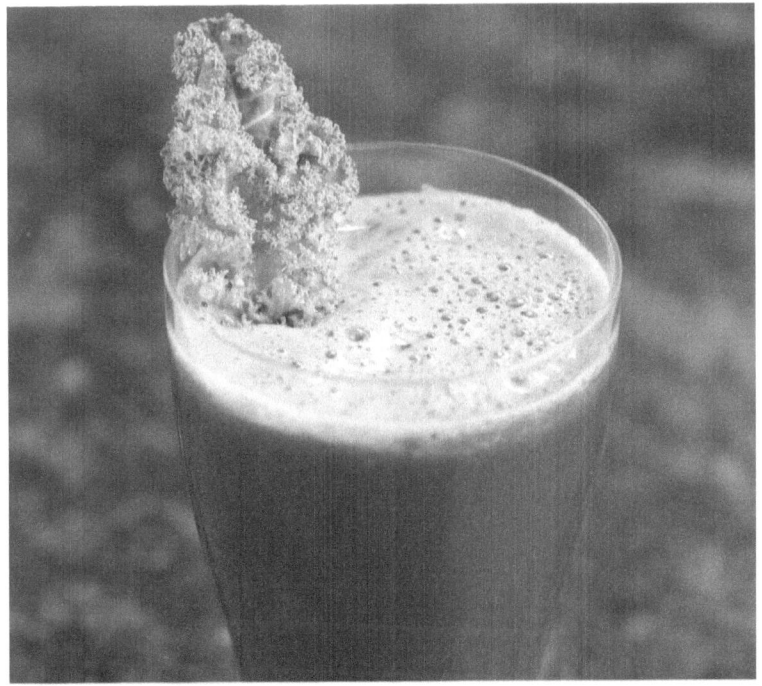

Chocked full of nutrition!

Serving Size: 1 serving

Ingredient List:

- 2 cups kale
- 2 pears

HHHHHHHHHHHHHHHHHHHHHHHHHHHHHHHHHHHHHHHH

Procedure:

1. Blend together kale and pears

Recipe 22: Crushed Pecan Zucchini Poppers

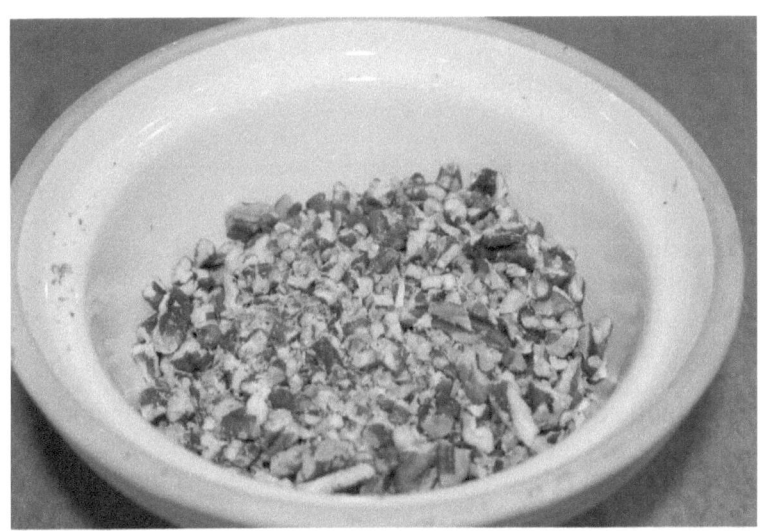

An excellent snack!

Serving Size: 8

Ingredient List:

- 8 1-2-inch-thick zucchini discs
- 2 egg whites
- 1 cup crushed pecans
- 2 teaspoons Italian seasoning

HHHHHHHHHHHHHHHHHHHHHHHHHHHHHHHHHHHHHHHH

Procedure:

1. Preheat oven to 425 and prepare baking tray

2. Combine crushed pecans and Italian seasoning; In another bowl beat egg whites; dip the discs into egg whites then toss in pecan crumbs; bake 15-20 minutes

Recipe 23: Twist of Melon Juice

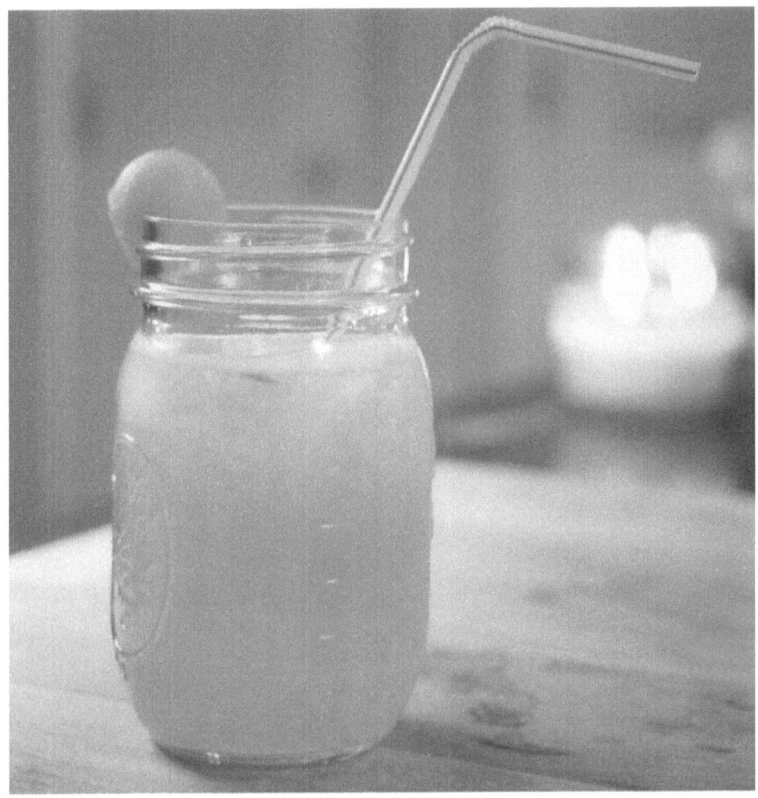

Substitute berries for the banana!

Serving Size: 1 serving

Ingredient List:

- 2 cups spinach
- 1/3 cup of watermelon juice
- ¼ cup banana juice

HHHHHHHHHHHHHHHHHHHHHHHHHHHHHHHHHHHHH

Procedure:

1. Blend spinach, watermelon, and banana together

Recipe 24: Asparagus, Beans, and Brown Rice

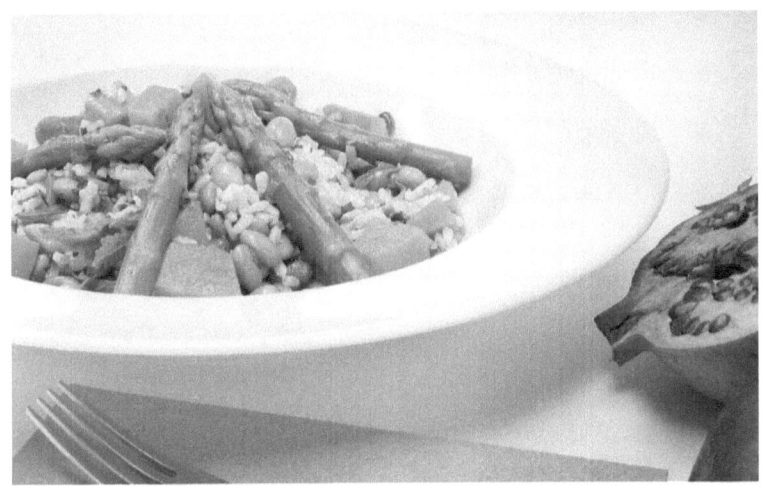

For an extra twist add avocado!

Serving Size: 1 9x9 dish

Ingredient List:

- 1 cup brown rice
- 2 cups alkaline water
- 1 cup worth asparagus spears
- 1 cup green beans
- Juice of 1 lemon
- Crushed pecans for topping

HHHHHHHHHHHHHHHHHHHHHHHHHHHHHHHHHHHHHHH

Procedure:

1. Preheat oven to 350 and prepare a 9x9 dish

2. Add rice, asparagus, beans; top with water, juice; sprinkle with crushed pecans; bake 30-35 minutes

Recipe 25: Avocado Kale Mixer

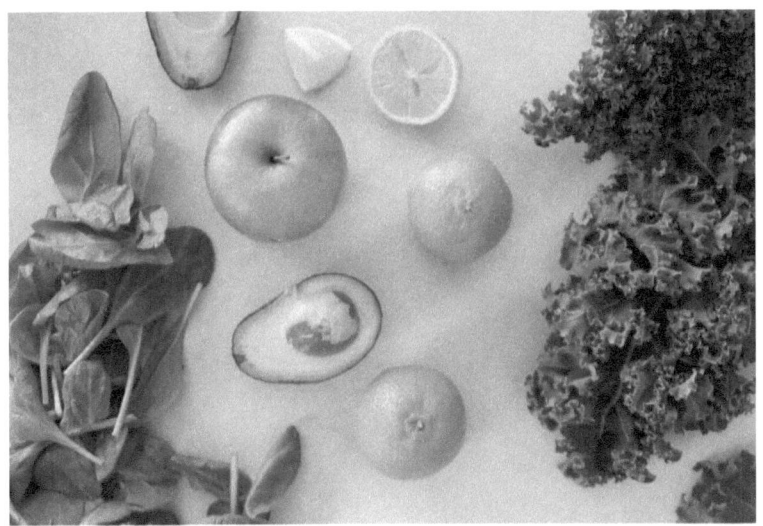

A favorite drink!

Serving Size: 1 serving

Ingredient List:

- Juice of 1 avocado
- 2 cups kale
- Juice of 1 apple

HHHHHHHHHHHHHHHHHHHHHHHHHHHHHHHHHHHHHHHH

Procedure:

1. Blend together avocado juice, kale, and apple juice

Recipe 26: Cauliflower Rice Egg Rolls

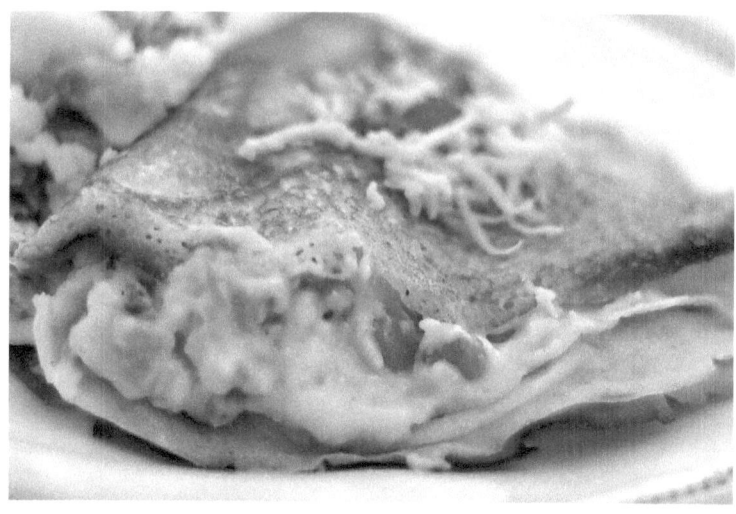

Cauliflower is a great substitute for meat!

Serving Size: 8 egg rolls

Ingredient List:

- 8 large egg roll wrappers
- 3 cups cauliflower rice
- 1 teaspoon 5 spice powder
- ½ cup finely diced or grated okra
- 2/3 cup cooked, drained, brown lentils
- ½ cup matchstick carrots
- ½ cup crumbled tofu

HHHHHHHHHHHHHHHHHHHHHHHHHHHHHHHHHHHHH

Procedure:

1. Preheat oven to 400 and prepare baking tray

2. Combine cauliflower rice, okra, lentils, carrots, crumbled tofu; mix in 5 spice powder; spoon into wrappers and fold as directed; bake 45 minutes

Recipe 27: Tofu Soup

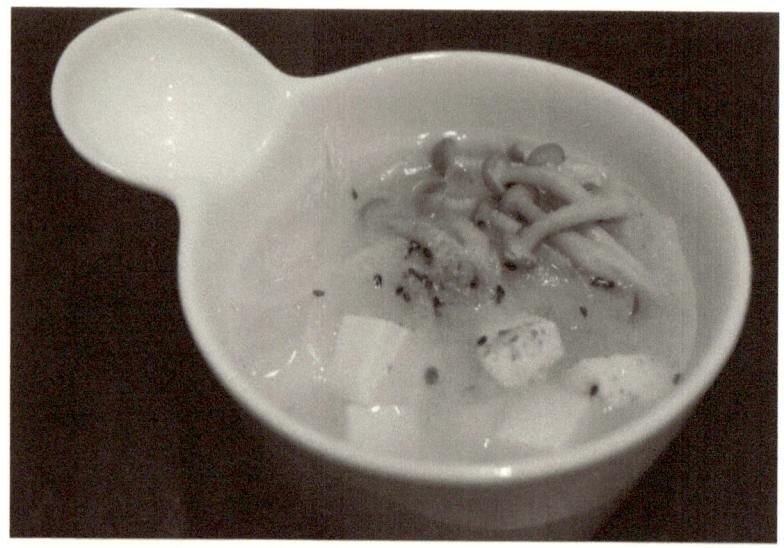

You'll love this simple tofu soup!

Serving Size: 1 serving

Ingredient List:

- Olive oil
- 2 cups firm, cubed, tofu
- 1/3 cup bell pepper trinity mix (diced mixture of red, yellow, green)
- 1 teaspoon EACH: cayenne powder, onion powder
- 4 oz. soba noodles
- 2 cups vegetable broth
- 1 teaspoon soy sauce
- ½ Tablespoons minced ginger

HHHHHHHHHHHHHHHHHHHHHHHHHHHHHHHHHHHHH

Procedure:

1. Cook soba noodles according to package directions; In a pot pour 1 to 2 teaspoons of olive oil brown tofu, peppers, cayenne powder, onion powder; add to vegetable broth, add soy sauce and ginger.

Recipe 28: Green Bean Casserole

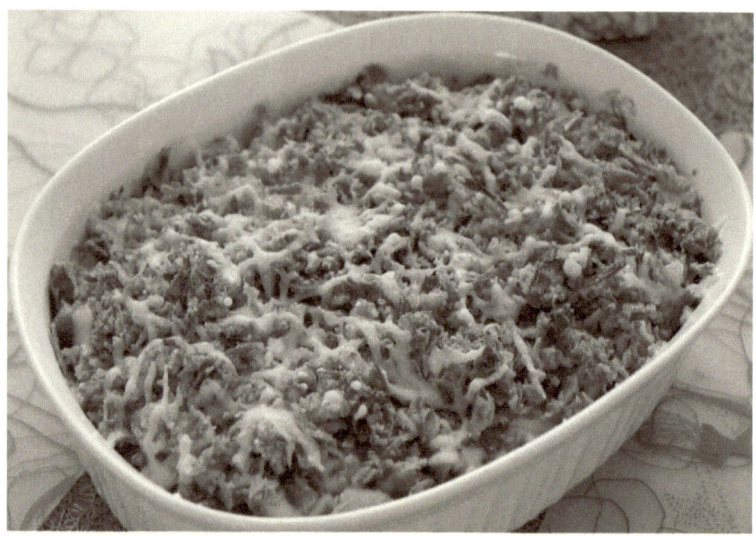

Delicious! Great over brown rice!

Serving Size: 1 9x9 dish

Ingredient List:

- 4 cups green beans
- 2 cups diced butternut squash
- 2 cup new baby potatoes
- 1-2 cup chopped or quartered tomatoes
- 3-4 cups water or vegetable broth

HHHHHHHHHHHHHHHHHHHHHHHHHHHHHHHHHHHHHH

Procedure:

1. Preheat oven to 350 and prepare a 9x9 dish

2. Mix together green beans, butternut squash, potatoes, and tomatoes; add liquids; bake 30-35 minutes

Recipe 29: Sweet Potato Wraps

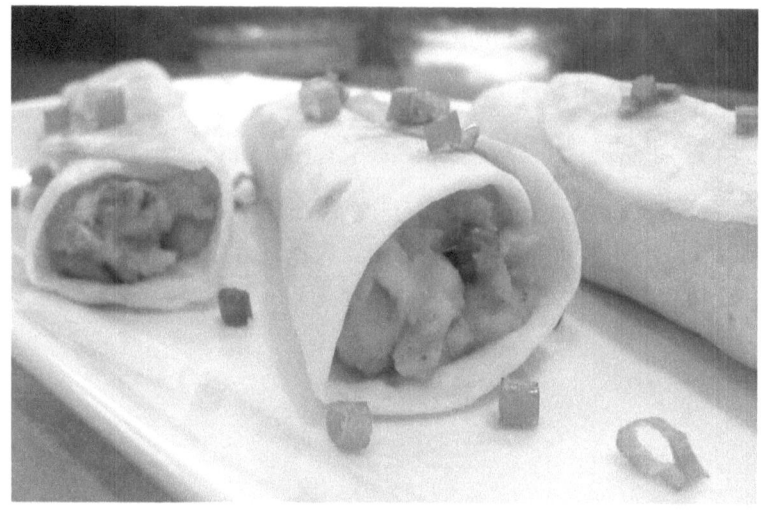

Great for brunch!

Serving Size: 1 serving

Ingredient List:

- 1 8 or 10 inch sun dried tomato sandwich wrap
- 1 sweet potato chopped
- ½ shallot diced
- 1 cup chopped kale
- 2 Tablespoons raisins
- 2 Tablespoons pine nuts

HHHHHHHHHHHHHHHHHHHHHHHHHHHHHHHHHHHHHH

Procedure:

1. In small bowl mix together sweet potato chunks, chopped kale, diced shallots, raisins, pine nuts; spoon into wrap

Recipe 30: Butter Beans

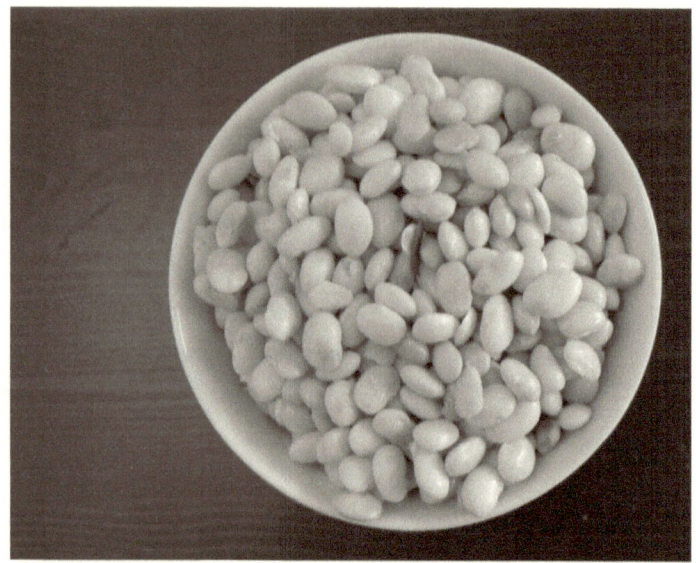

Great on cool days!

Serving Size: 3-4 servings

Ingredient List:

- 1 diced red onion
- 4 cups butter beans
- 6 cups water
- 2 cups kale or spinach
- ½ teaspoons cayenne powder

HHHHHHHHHHHHHHHHHHHHHHHHHHHHHHHHHHHHHHH

Procedure:

1. In large pot or Dutch oven sauté onions 3-5 minutes, pour in beans and water; bring to a boil, reduce heat, let simmer 5-6 hours; about 30 minutes before finished add spinach or kale and cayenne powder

Recipe 31: Salad Wrap

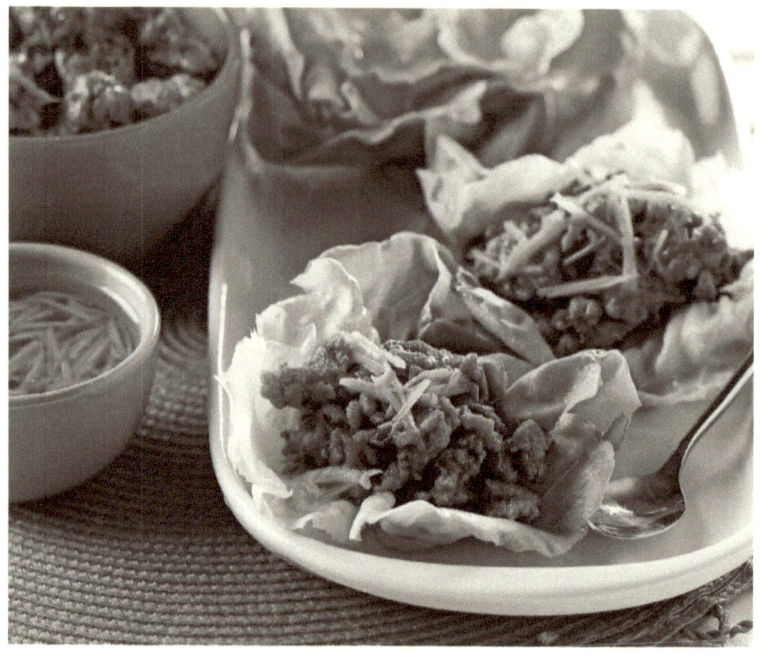

Take your salad on the go!

Serving Size: 1 serving

Ingredient List:

- 1 8 or 10-inch spinach wrap
- 2 large leaves of iceberg or romaine lettuce
- 1 cucumber cut into strips lengthwise
- 3 slices of tomato
- 1 yellow bell pepper cut into strips or ½ cup banana peppers
- ½ block firm, cubed tofu blackened
- 1/3 cup almond slivers (optional)

HHHHHHHHHHHHHHHHHHHHHHHHHHHHHHHHHHHHHHH

Procedure:

1. Layout wrap, layer with lettuce, cucumber, tomato slices, yellow bell pepper, blackened tofu, almonds

Recipe 32: Carrot Broccoli Salad

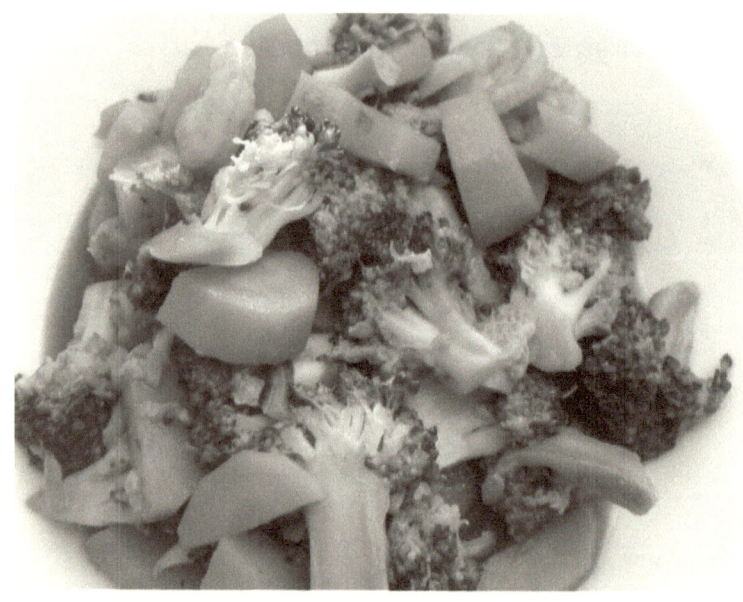

Great as a side or alone!

Serving Size: 4 servings

Ingredient List:

- 2 cups matchstick carrots
- 2 cups grated broccoli
- 1 tablespoon minced garlic
- 2 cups chopped leeks
- Juice of 1 lemon
- Diced parsley or basil

HHHHHHHHHHHHHHHHHHHHHHHHHHHHHHHHHHHHHHH

Procedure:

1. In bowl mix together carrots, broccoli, garlic, leek, basil or parsley; pour juice over salad; keep refrigerated in air tight container

Recipe 33: Simple Oatmeal Smoothie

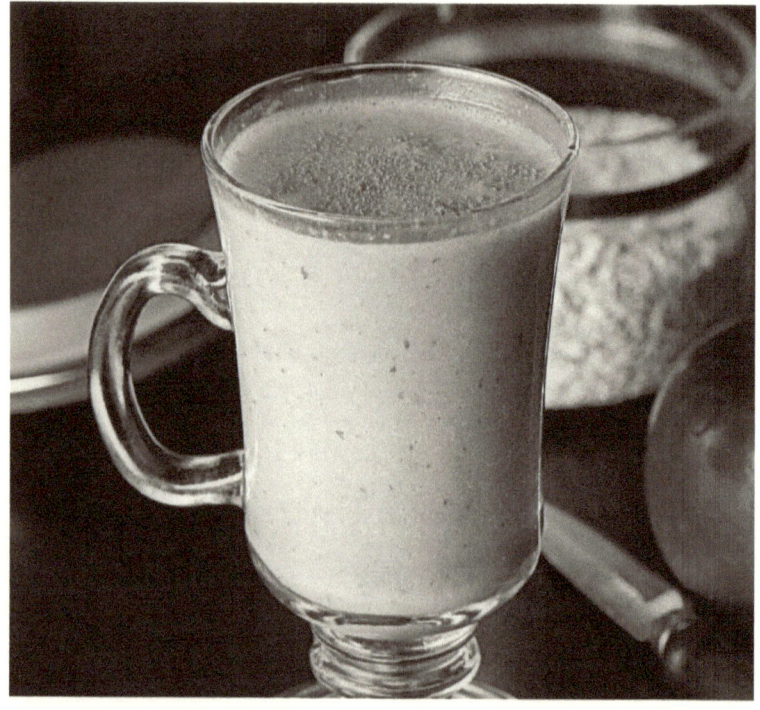

Make ahead of time, will keep 3-5 days in refrigerator!

Serving Size: 1 serving

Ingredient List:

- ½ cup oats
- 1 cup almond milk
- ½ cup blueberries
- 1 teaspoon honey

HHHHHHHHHHHHHHHHHHHHHHHHHHHHHHHHHHHHHHH

Procedure:

1. Blend together oats, milk, blueberries, honey

Recipe 34: Roasted Cauliflower Casserole

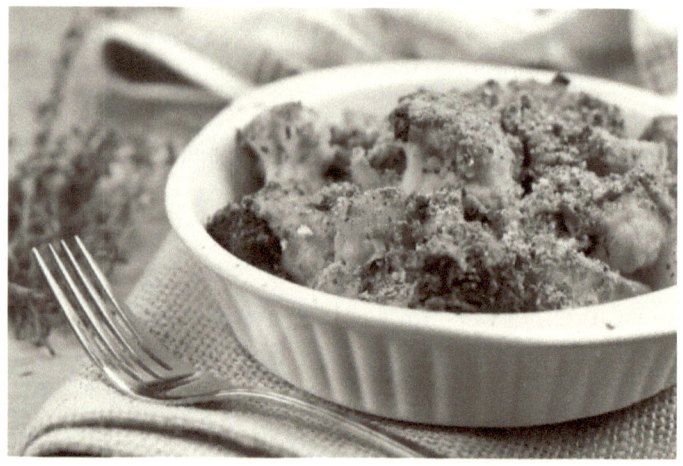

Great dish to introduce skeptics to the alkaline diet!

Serving Size: 1 9x9 dish

Ingredient List:

- 1 tablespoon coconut oil
- 1 head of cauliflower, cut a washed
- 1 chopped sweet potatoes, washed and dried
- ½ diced stalk of celery
- ½ cup caramelized shallot

HHHHHHHHHHHHHHHHHHHHHHHHHHHHHHHHHHHHHHHH

Procedure:

1. Preheat oven to 400 and prepare 9x9 dish

2. Place prepared cauliflower and sweet potatoes in dish and toss in oil; in skillet sauté celery and onions 2-4 minutes; place on top of cauliflower and sweet potatoes; cook 30-40 minutes

Recipe 35: Brown Sugar Oatmeal Bars

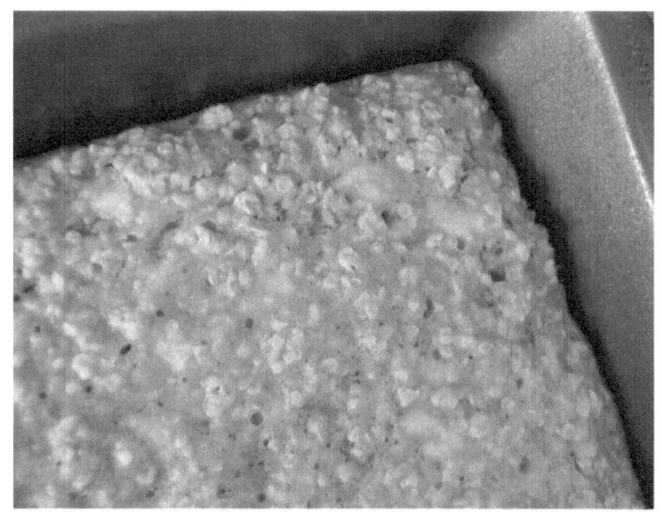

Ingredient List:

- 1 cup old fashion oats
- 1 cup almond flour
- 2 egg whites
- 1 stick clarified butter, 8 Tablespoons
- 1 cup packed browned sugar
- ½ cup raisins
- Honey, for drizzling on top, optional

HHHHHHHHHHHHHHHHHHHHHHHHHHHHHHHHHHHHHHH

Procedure:

1. Preheat oven to 350 and prepare 9x9 cooking dish

2. In bowl combine oats, flour and set aside; cream together clarified butter and egg whites; Mix in brown sugar to butter mixture; Slowly add flour mix to butter mix; stir in raisins; pour into dish

Recipe 36: Coconut Sweet Potato Wedges

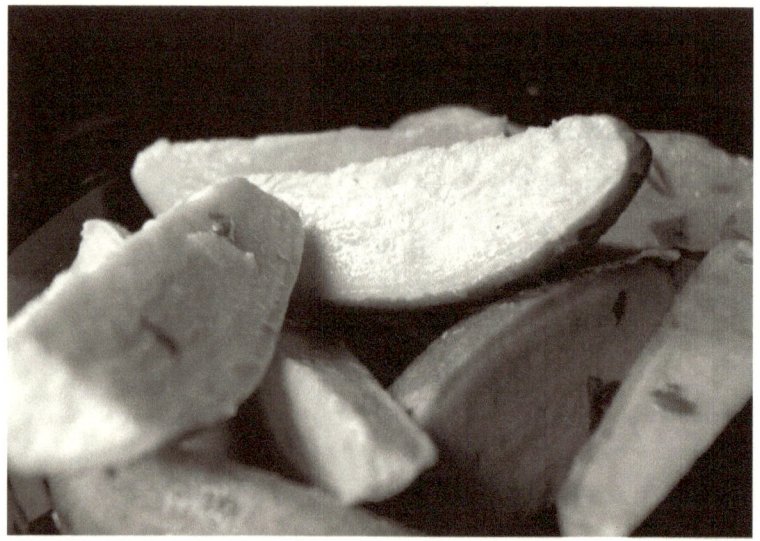

You'll love these!

Serving Size: 1 9x9 dish

Ingredient List:

- 1 sweet potato cut into wedges
- 1/3 – ½ cup coconut oil
- Black pepper or red pepper flakes

Procedure:

1. Preheat oven to 400 and prepare a 9x9 casserole dish

2. Place wedges in dish, toss in oil, sprinkle with pepper; cook 20 - 25 minutes

Recipe 37: Banana Cherry Crockpot Oats

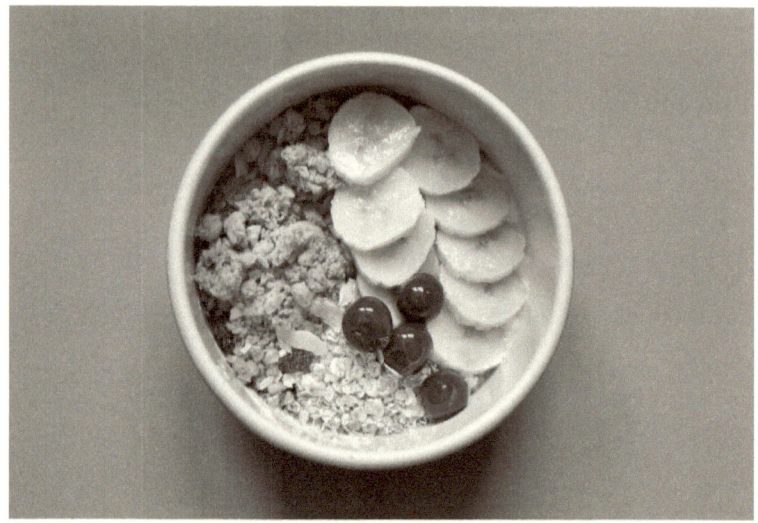

These will keep you coming back for more!

Serving Size: 1 serving

Ingredient List:

- 1 cups oats- old fashioned
- 5-6 cups of water
- ½ cup milk
- 2 sliced or mashed bananas
- ½ cup cherries and juice

HHHHHHHHHHHHHHHHHHHHHHHHHHHHHHHHHHHHH

Procedure:

1. Place oats, water, milk, bananas, cherries into crockpot chamber and cook on low overnight, 8 hours.

Recipe 38: Zucchini Poppers

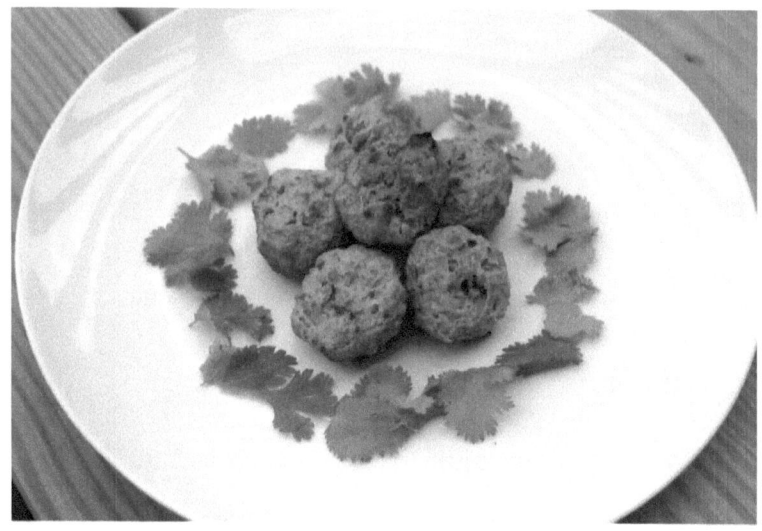

Make a bunch, they are addictive!

Serving Size: 12-15 poppers

Ingredient List:

- 12-15 1-inch disc shaped slices of zucchini
- 2 beaten egg white
- 1 cup flour
- 1/3 cup shredded parmesan cheese (optional)
- 1/3 cup crushed pecans

HHHHHHHHHHHHHHHHHHHHHHHHHHHHHHHHHHHHHHHH

Procedure:

1. Preheat oven to 425 and prepare baking tray

2. Dip zucchini slices into egg then in flour mixed with cheese and pecans; cook 20-30 minutes at 425

Recipe 39: Trinity Quinoa

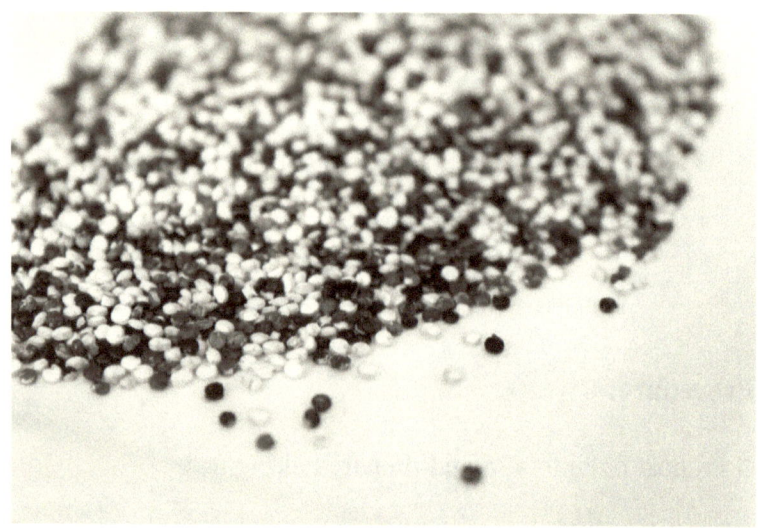

Great as a side or on its own!

Serving Size: 1 serving

Ingredient List:

- 1 cup quinoa
- 2 cups water
- ½ teaspoons Italian seasoning
- ½ cup trinity mix (diced celery, onion, and garlic)

HHHHHHHHHHHHHHHHHHHHHHHHHHHHHHHHHHHHHH

Procedure:

1. In dish let quinoa sit in water until it soaks it up then cook as directed on package, add seasoning and trinity mix

Recipe 40: Salmon and Veggie Stew

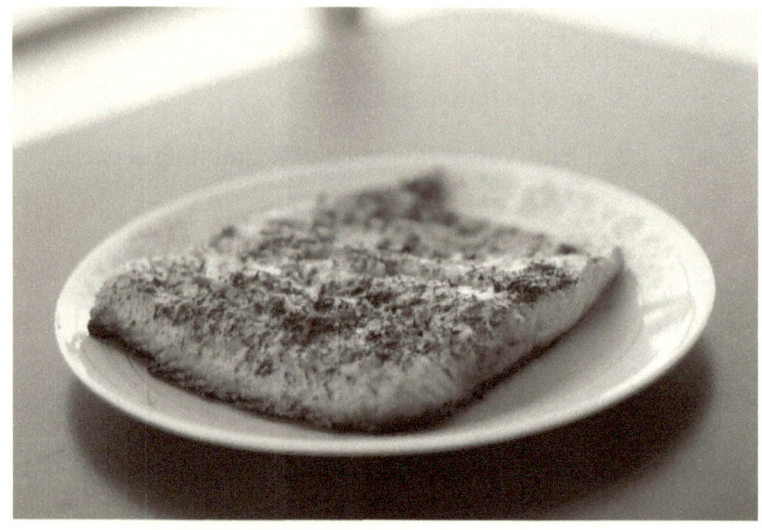

Great for various types of seafood!

Serving Size: 2 servings (2 filets, approx. 3-4 cups of stew)

Ingredient List:

- 1 tablespoon olive oil
- 1 teaspoon celery salt, pepper, garlic powder
- 2 ½ cups vegetable broth
- 1/3 cup baby carrots
- 5-7 broccoli florets
- ½ cup corn
- ½ cup diced potatoes
- ¼ cup mix of onion soup seasoning (like Lipton's)
- 2 filets of salmon

HHHHHHHHHHHHHHHHHHHHHHHHHHHHHHHHHHHHHHH

Procedure:

1. In Dutch oven mix together: oil, onion soup mix, celery salt, pepper, garlic powder, carrots, broccoli, corn, potatoes, and broth; bring to boil, reduce, let simmer 35-45 minutes; In skillet cook salmon 3-5 minutes per side

Recipe 41: Kale Spring Rolls

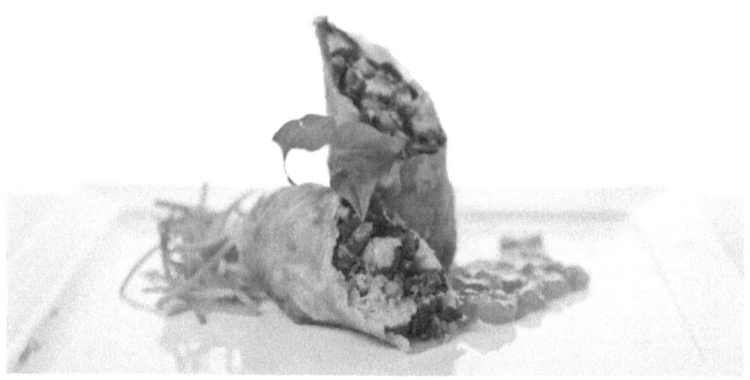

Cream cheese is mildly acidic so have these as an occasional treat!

Serving Size: 5-7 spring rolls

Ingredient List:

- 4-6 cups kale leaves
- 2-3 blocks cream cheese
- 1 can, washed, cannellini or garbanzo beans
- 5-7 spring roll wrappers

HHHHHHHHHHHHHHHHHHHHHHHHHHHHHHHHHHHHHH

Procedure:

1. Cream together kale and cream cheese; stir in beans; spoon into spring roll wrappers; bake at 425 for 20-30 minutes or fry

Recipe 42: Tofu Hummus

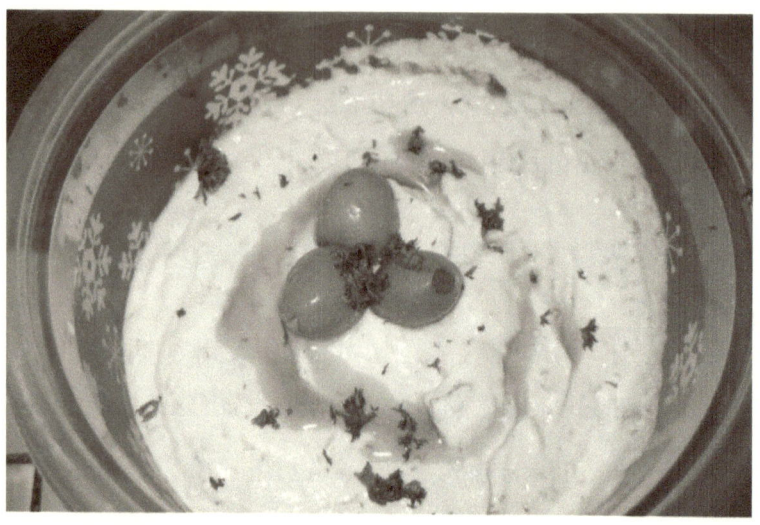

Also go great with homemade tortilla chips!

Serving Size: approx. 2-3 cups

Ingredient List:

- 1 can, rinsed and drained, garbanzo beans
- ½ cup crumbled silken tofu
- 1 diced purple onion
- ½ teaspoons garlic powder
- 1 teaspoon lemon juice
- 1 teaspoon oregano

HHHHHHHHHHHHHHHHHHHHHHHHHHHHHHHHHHHHHHH

Procedure:

1. Blend tofu, beans, onion, garlic powder, lemon juice, and oregano

Recipe 43: Summer Fruit Salad

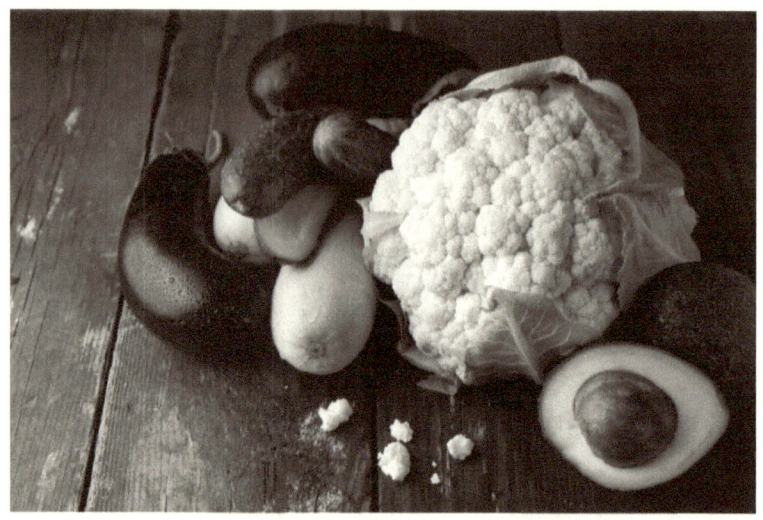

Ingredient List:

- ½ honeydew melon
- 1 diced cucumber
- 1 diced avocado
- 2 tablespoon pistachios
- 1 cup roasted red peppers
- thyme

HHHHHHHHHHHHHHHHHHHHHHHHHHHHHHHHHHHHHHH

Procedure:

1. Mix together melon, cucumber, avocado, pistachios, peppers; sprinkle with thyme

Recipe 44: Tortilla chips with Avocado Dip

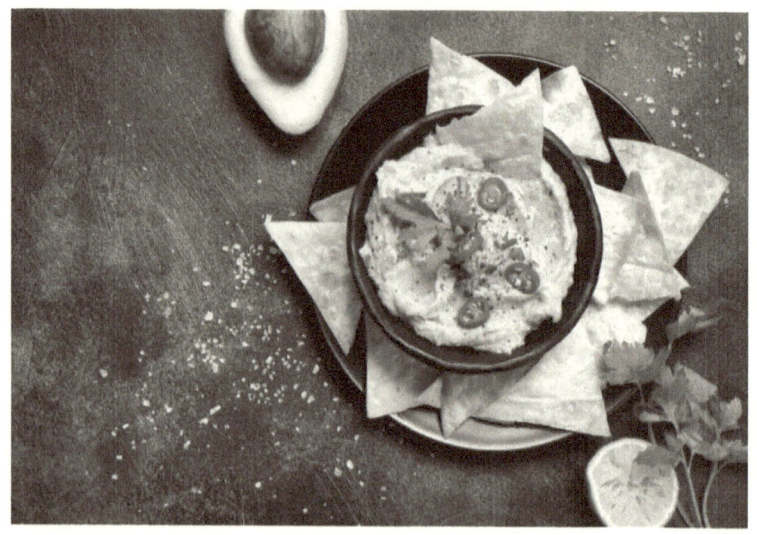

Quick and easy!

Serving Size: 12-16 chips and approx. 1- 1 ½ cup dip

Ingredient List:

- 3-4 corn tortillas
- Garlic powder with chopped parsley for sprinkling
- olive oil spray
- 1 diced avocado
- 1 teaspoon lemon juice
- 1 teaspoon diced cilantro (optional)
- ½ cup diced red roasted peppers

HHHHHHHHHHHHHHHHHHHHHHHHHHHHHHHHHHHHHHH

Procedure:

1. Preheat oven to 425 and prepare baking tray

2. Cut tortillas into triangles; spread out on baking sheet; sprinkle with garlic powder and parsley; spray with olive oil; Cook 8-10 minutes. 3. Puree avocado pieces along with lemon juice; stir in cilantro and red pepper. Refrigerate until served

Recipe 45: Flatbread Pizza with a Tomato Based Sauce

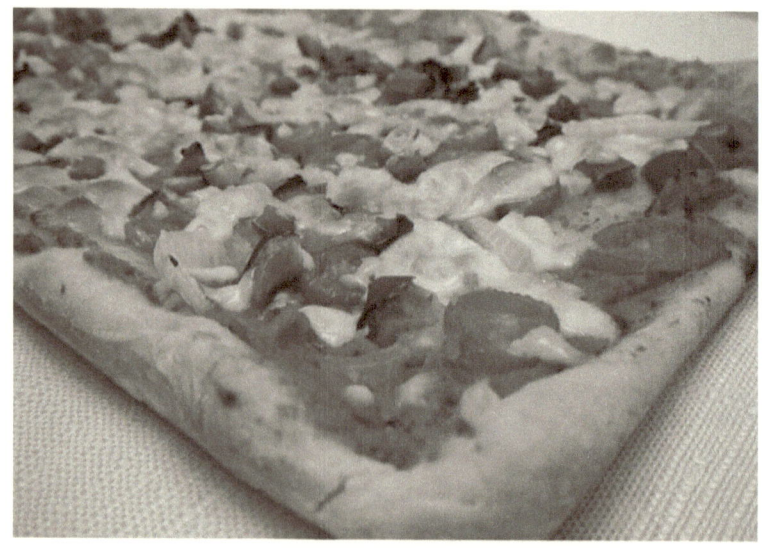

Ingredient List:

- 1 piece of flatbread

Sauce:

- 4-6 cherry tomatoes
- 1 teaspoon olive oil
- ½ Tablespoons honey or agave
- 1 teaspoon Italian seasoning
- 1 tablespoon water (if more is needed add by ½ Tablespoons to help thin out sauce)

Toppings:

- ½ cup crumbled tofu
- 1 cup fajita style onions and peppers
- 1 cup spinach
- ½ pack, washed and sliced baby shiitake mushrooms

HHHHHHHHHHHHHHHHHHHHHHHHHHHHHHHHHHHHHH

Procedure:

1. Place washed cherry tomatoes, oil, honey/agave, seasoning, water in food processor and puree; spread onto flatbread; top with tofu, onions and peppers, spinach, mushrooms; bake as directed on package

Recipe 46: Pineapple Coconut Popsicles

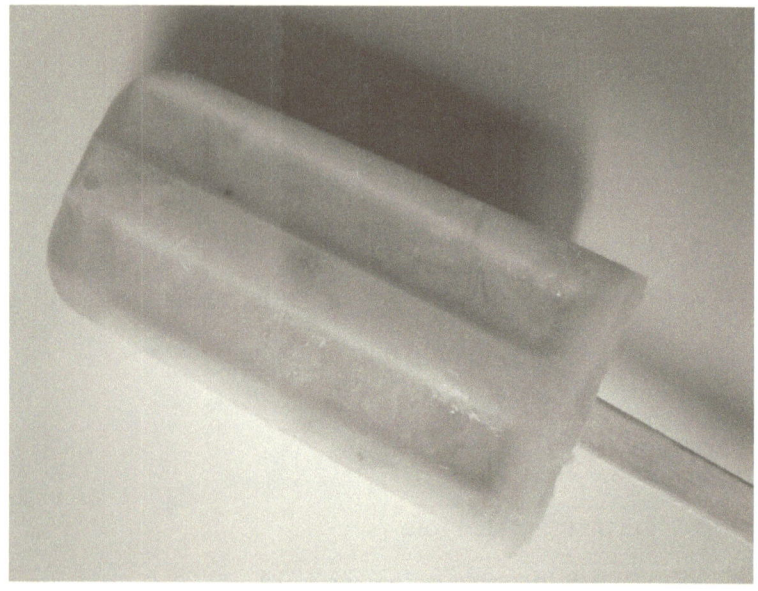

Very flavorful!

Serving Size: 4-6

Ingredient List:

- 1 cup coconut milk
- 2 cups pineapple juice

HHHHHHHHHHHHHHHHHHHHHHHHHHHHHHHHHHHHHHH

Procedure:

1. Mix together coconut milk and pineapple juice; pour into popsicle molds

Recipe 47: Spring Pizza with Avocado Sauce

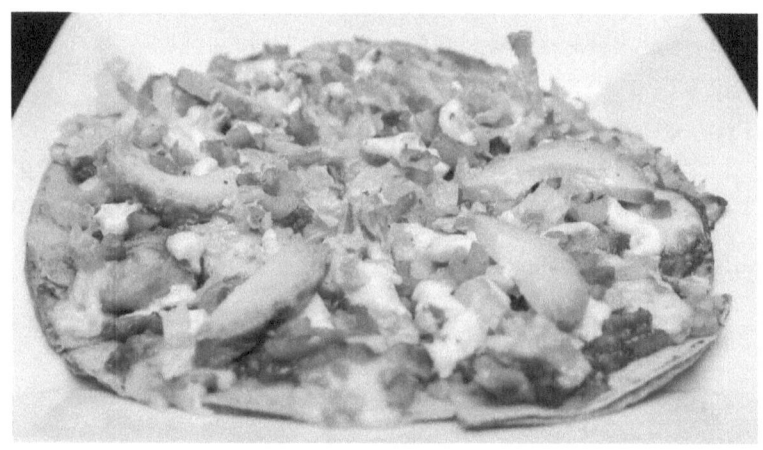

Perfect for those who like big flavor!

Serving Size: 1 pizza

Ingredient List:

- 1 shell, package, or homemade crust (see recipe below)

Sauce:

- 2-3 avocados chopped
- 1 teaspoon lemon juice
- ½ teaspoons chili powder
- ½ teaspoons jalapeno powder
- ½ teaspoons onion powder

HHHHHHHHHHHHHHHHHHHHHHHHHHHHHHHHHHHHHHH

Procedure:

1. Place avocados, lemon juice, chili powder, jalapeno powder, and onion powder in blender and puree; spread onto pizza crust

Toppings:

- Strips of red pepper
- Strips of purple onion
- ½ pack washed and sliced button mushrooms
- Crumbled tofu

HHHHHHHHHHHHHHHHHHHHHHHHHHHHHHHHHHHHHHHH

Procedure:

2. Bake according to package directions

Recipe 48: Almond Berry Popsicles

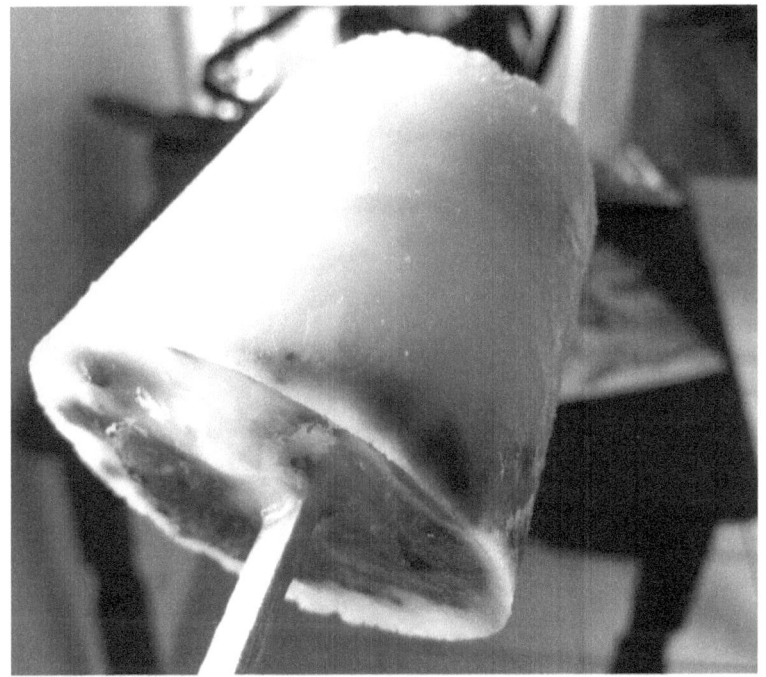

A great summer treat!

Serving Size: 4-6

Ingredient List:

- 1 cup almond milk
- 1 cups apple juice
- ½ cup strawberry juice

HHHHHHHHHHHHHHHHHHHHHHHHHHHHHHHHHHHHHH

Procedure:

1. Mix all liquids together and pour into popsicle molds; freeze 1 hour

Recipe 49: Alkaline Pizza Dough

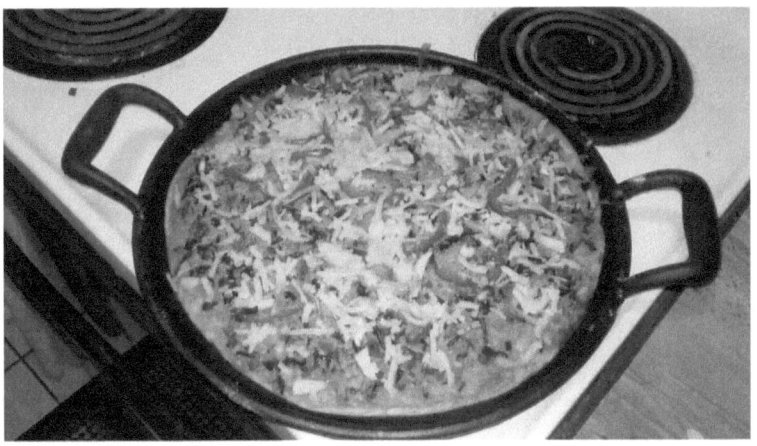

Use this recipe as a base for all of your dough needs!

Serving Size: 1 10x8 sheet of dough

Ingredient List:

- 1 ½ cups almond flour
- 1 cup alkaline or spring water
- 1 teaspoon onion powder
- ½ teaspoons sea salt

HHHHHHHHHHHHHHHHHHHHHHHHHHHHHHHHHHHHHHHH

Procedure:

1. Mix together flour, water, onion powder, sea salt; roll out dough and place on a baking sheet; bake 5 minutes in 400 degrees oven before spreading sauce on

Recipe 50: Nutty Tomato Treats

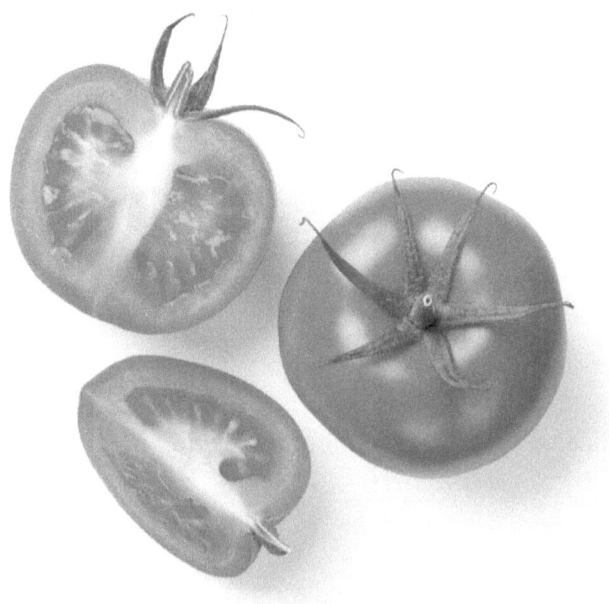

Always a big hit at potlucks!

Serving Size: 10-12 Treats

Ingredient List:

- 2 beefsteak tomatoes cut into 1-inch discs
- 1 tablespoon coconut or olive oil
- 1 cup breadcrumbs
- 1 teaspoon Italian seasoning
- ½ cup crushed almonds or pistachios

HHHHHHHHHHHHHHHHHHHHHHHHHHHHHHHHHHHHHHHH

Procedure:

1. Preheat oven to 350 and prepare baking tray

2. Mix together breadcrumbs, seasoning, and nuts; toss tomato slices in oil lightly coating front and back; dip slices in mixture; layout on tray and cook 45 minutes

About the Author

Jennifer Jones is an accomplished chef, devoted wife and loving mother of two who lives in Boulder, Colorado. As head chef at one of Colorado's most exclusive restaurants, Jennifer's culinary prowess has become legendary and she is often called over to the tables of the rich and famous to accept deep praise for her work.

The beautiful scenery of Boulder is often used as inspiration for some of Jennifer's artistically decorated dishes and the praise is just as much for her creative presentation as the exquisite taste of her food. Her use of greenery to bring out the delectable cuts of meat and fish that adorn the dinner plates is no less than a work of art, and she describes herself as an artist and not a chef.

Jones flourished under the mentorship of her professor at August Escoffier Culinary School of the Arts and went on to study at the Cordon Bleu to perfect her repertoire of international cuisine. While studying abroad, she kept close contact with her mentor from Escoffier, eventually marrying him when she came back to North America.

With all of that culinary ability, you would think some would rub off on the kids? Jennifer's two daughters are both excellent chefs in their own right and have plans to attend Escoffier like their parents. A culinary dynasty, perhaps?

Author's Afterthoughts

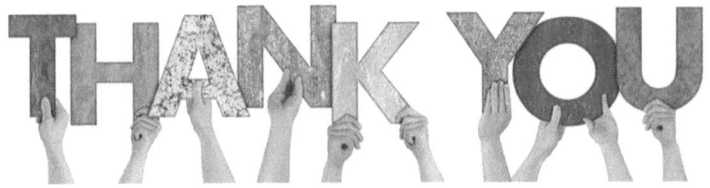

With so many books out there to choose from, I want to thank you for choosing this one and taking precious time out of your life to buy and read my work. Readers like you are the reason I take such passion in creating these books.

It is with gratitude and humility that I express how honored I am to become a part of your life and I hope that you take the same pleasure in reading this book as I did in writing it.

Can I ask one small favour? I ask that you write an honest and open review on Amazon of what you thought of the book. This will help other readers make an informed choice on whether to buy this book.

Sincerely,

Jennifer Jones

If you want to be the first to know about news, new books, events and giveaways, subscribe to my newsletter by clicking the link below

https://Jennifer-Jones.gr8.com

or Scan QR-code

www.ingramcontent.com/pod-product-compliance
Lightning Source LLC
Chambersburg PA
CBHW031325290526
45784CB00014B/1508